Secretes Revealed,

STAY YOUNG and HEALTHY

with LIMITLESS ENERGY

Discover Amazing Nutrients That Energizes

Protect your heart, brain and body

Prevent Heart Attacks and Strokes

Feel Young and Energetic Like a Kid

Dr. Arta Tran Dash, M.Sc., M. S., Ph. D.

Retired Professor

LOKA SAMASTA SUKHINO BHABANTU

(Let Each And Every Person In The Universe Be Hale and Hearty)

VEDAS

DEDICATION

This book is dedicated to the memory of my father (Linga Raj Dash) and my mother (Mukta Debi), whose unconditional love nurtured my life through and through.

It is also dedicated to all those who read it, use it, and benefit from it.

DISCLAIMER

This book is not intended to diagnose, treat or replace the service of a doctor. If you have any health conditions or are under a doctor's care, you must consult your physician or a healthcare professional before you apply any of the recommendations set forth in the pages of this book.

All information available in this book is for educational purposes only, and none of the stated products have been FDA approved. Any application of the recommendations mentioned in this book is at the readers' discretion and sole risk.

The publication is offered "as is" without warranty of any kind either expressed or implied, including but not limited to, the implied warranties of merchantability, suitability for a particular purpose or non-infringement. Descriptions of or reference to products or publications does not imply endorsement of that product or publication.

Here is how you can use the information in this book to improve your health and wellness. Being Empowered with these powerful armies of information, and the knowledge gathered from it, you would be able to discuss your health problems with a healthcare professional and design a regimen that is conducive to your health and well being, instead of just being drugged to death and suffer from lethal side effects of these drugs, causing serious debilitating, chronic diseases.

If you find your physician is unwilling to discuss the issue, find another physician or a healthcare professional that is more sensitive to your wish and willing to take the time to listen to you for your well being. You need to know all your options before embarking on a particular regimen or a procedure.

TABLE OF CONTENTS

After Heart Attack

Heart Failure

Heart Surgery

Guarding the brain after cardiac arrest

Help slow neurodegenerative disease progression

Slows the progression of Macular degeneration

Chapter Four

How CoQ10 Help Fight Cancer

Mitochondria (power of cells)

Free radicals (lethal chemicals)

Cardiovascular health and brain health

Chemotherapy drugs (anthracyclines & anddrialmycine)

Cardiotoxicity, cardiomyo[athy

Immune system cells

Immunostimulatory effect of CoQ10

Oncology

Chapter Five

Brain and Heart Need PQQ

Super Star Nutrient PQQ

Telomere is the bits of DNA at the end of each chromosome

Mitochondria—tiny power plants in each cell

Mitochondrial DNA complex

Grow new mitochondria

Chapter Six

As Your Mitochondria Disappear, So Does Your Life Force

Pyroloquinoline quinine (PQQ)

Nerve Growth Factor

Excitotoxicity

Replicate

Mitochondrial formation

Nerve growth factor (NGF)

Memory, cognition, and learning

Chapter Seven

Healthy Brains Need Healthy Mitochondria

Energy hungry organ

Heart and brain

Mitochondria decay

Neurodegenerative diseases

Alzheimer's, Parkinson's and dementia

Apoptosis or cell suicide

Neurological and brain disorders

Ischemic stroke

Chapter Eight

PQQ Inhibits Malformed Brain Proteins

Malformed protein

Beta amyloid

Alpha – synuelein

Alzheimer's and Parkinson's

Chapter Nine

PQQ Prevents Glucose-Induced Brain Damage

Neurological damage

Alzheimer's is type - 3 diabetes

Male fertility and sperm motility

Cells' energy factories

ATP energy (Adenosine triphosphate)

Power generators

Chapter Ten

PQQ Induces Cancer Cell Death

Tumor cells apoptosis

Promonocytic leukemia U937 and lymphoma EL-4 cells

Microscopic energy factories

Balance of cell life and cell death

Cell suicide is programmed into your genes

Cycle of life

Chapter Eleven

Where is it found the most?

Power centers of your body

Heart, brain, liver, kidneys, pancreas

Parsley, green tea, papaya, kiwi, apple orange

Carrot, celery, spinach, legumes, pava beans, peanuts

SIRT1 genes

Resveratrol, Alpha Lipoic Acid

Introduction: Drench your body in boundless energy with

Two Amazing Nutrients CoQ10 and PQQ

Stay Healthy and Young with Unlimited Energy even into Your Golden Years

If you want to stay youthful and have all the benefits and power of youth as long as possible, it is imperative to learn about two very remarkable natural nutrients, Coenzyme Q10 (CoQ10) and PQQ (Pyrroloquinoline quinine.)

Coernzyme Q10 (CoQ10) is a nutrient found in every cell in your body. Your body makes CoQ10. Your cells use tt to produce energy your body needs for cell growth and maintenance. Your CoQ10 levels decline as you age. Take CoQ10 supplements to replenish the levels of deficiency of CoQ10. CoQ10 helps maintain healthy blood pressure and cholesterol levels, promotes arterial health and support strong heartbeats

Your hearts beats around 100,000 times a day; in order to function properly it needs the nutrient CoQ10. CoQ10 is considered heart tonic, often referred to as spark plug. When CoQ10 levels get low, your heart suffers a lot under strain to do its job. Ultimately your entire body suffers.

Clinical studies have linked significantly decreased levels of CoQ10 to a wide variety of diseases. Because the enzyme CoQ10 is in high concentration in heart muscle cells, deficiency has been linked to cardiovascular diseases, including angina, arrhythmia, and heart failure.

Problems, such as blood sugar regulation, gum disease, and stomach ulcer have also been linked to CoQ10 deficiency. Many pharmaceutical drugs like statins (cholesterol lowering drugs) deplete CoQ10. It is essential to supplement CoQ10 to replenish the level.

There are many more health benefits of CoQ10 like improved immune system, heart muscle cells, effective in the treatment of angina, atherosclerosis, male fertility, sperm count and sperm motility, mitral valve, muscular dystrophy, fight cancer and so on. KEEP READING.

We learned from above that heart needs CoQ10. Now we will learn from below that Brain needs PQQ

Mitochondria: *The source of life in your body*

Mitochondria are tiny power plants or power house inside each cell. Mitochondria are the only power plants or microscopic energy factories inside your cells. Mitochondria are the only power plants inside each cell. They are so critical they have their own DNA and that's what connects them to telomeres (bits of DNA at the end of chromosome.)

Thus, they can **REPLICATE.** They replicate independently of the cell in which they reside. This means mitochondrial replication is not coupled to cell division. Thus, they INCRESE numbers within a cell, if they have the right nutrient. This nutrient is PQQ, Pyroloquinoline quinine. Researchers proved that PQQ produce **new mitochondria**, and also **repairs** the damaged ones.

Recent clinical studies reveal that your brain is a prime target for mitochondrial decay more than any other organs in your body. This is because of the high-energy demands of your brain cells, and their exposer to large amounts of oxygen makes them vulnerable to damage from free radicals and oxidative stress.

If the damage is too severe, the brain cells trigger the destruction of their own mitochondria. Fewer mitochondria in your brain cells mean you lose your ability to make energy and your mental performance decline.

Ultimately, this causes your brain cells commit "**cell Suicide or apoptosis.**" This loss of cells in your brain tissue affects your **mobility**, your ability to **learn**, and your **memor**y, leading **to all kinds of neurological and brain disorders.**

Fortunately we have PQQ to the rescue.

Unfortunately, mitochondria die off as we get older. **As your mitochondria disappear, so does your life source.** Fortunately PQQ comes to the rescue. PQQ not only grows new mitochondria, but also repairs the damaged ones; and also improves the efficacy of the existing ones

PQQ is neuroproctive and has a restorative and rejuvenating impact on your brain. it triggers the growth of brand new nerve cells and brand new brain cells. PQQ can play a vital role in preventing brain from ravages of strokes. In clinical studies, it was shown that PQQ reduced ischemic stroke damage potentially improving quality of life following a stroke.

Other benefits of PQQ, to name a few:

- helps increase sperm motility, improving male fertility
- induces cancer cell death
- Prevents Glucose-Induced Brain Damage
- Prevents Alzheimer's and Parkinson's diseases

The key to staying young and healthy is having MORE mitochondria that are healthy enough to produce energy.

Remember, the more of these power generators you have, the more you'll feel like that energetic 5-year-old who never seems to run out of steam

Therefore, when you combine PQQ with CoQ10, amazing things can happen.

Doses: 100 mg Ubiquinol and 10 mg PQQ in the morning, and 100 mg ubiquinol in the evening

You can find these nutrients in any of your local Health Food Stores.

Chapter One

Your Heart Needs CoQ10

CoQ10 Fuel Your Heart

Coernzyme Q10 (CoQ10)

CoQ10 is a nutrient found in every cell in your body. Your body makes CoQ10. Your cells use tt to produce energy your body needs for cell growth and maintenance. It also functions as a powerful antioxidant which protects the body from damage caused by lethal free radicals. A free radical is a molecule with unpaired atoms or missing an atom that make it highly unstable. As a result, they start attacking healthy cells to steal their atoms, and make them unstable. When enough of the cells are damaged – it may cause heart attacks, strokes, cancer, and other chronic diseases.

Free radicals can damage cell membranes, alter DNA code and even cell death. Free radicals can also cause premature aging as well as myriads of health problems, including heart disease, strokes, cancer. Antioxidants like CoQ10 hunt for free radicals and neutralize them and help prevent some of the damages they might have cause.

Your CoQ10 levels decline as you age. Take CoQ10 supplements to replenish the levels of deficiency of CoQ10. CoQ10 helps maintain healthy blood pressure and cholesterol levels, promotes arterial health and support strong heartbeats. The other proven health benefits are – gum, brain and skin. Studies indicate that it may help prevent migraines and slow hearing loss.

Your heart beats around 100,000 times a day; in order to function properly it needs the nutrient CoQ10. CoQ10 is considered heart tonic, often referred to as spark plug. CoQ10 is responsible for **converting carbs and fat into ATP energy**, the energy desperately needed by your

- Heart
- Brain
- All of your cells
- It effectively destroys the age--robbing free radicals
  Which are known to damage cells and cause cell death
- CoQ10 maintain youthful mitochondrial (cell's energy factories) activity
- Mitochondrial dysfunction is linked to accelerated aging
- CoQ10 energizes every cells in the body and enhances mitochondrial
  Function

Coenzyme Q10 is a mitochondrial energizer that has shown remarkable effects against common heart ailments and neurological disorders

Without CoQ10, heart cells would not be able to produce energy fuel ATP (adenosine triphosphate). Your heart suffers when there is deficiency of nutrient CoQ10. Many scientific research studies have shown that CoQ10 lend powerful support for your entire cardiovascular system. Moreover, your mitochondria (cells' tiny power plants) need CoQ10 to generate ATP energy to keep your heart cells functioning and healthy. When CoQ10 levels get low, your heart suffers a lot under strain to do its job. Ultimately your entire body suffers.

CoQ10 comes in **two forms**.

- **Ubiquinon:** this is sold widely in the market, and most people take this one. It is very vital for your health, since it powers up your heart, brain and vitality in the **intra cellular** regions of your body. Research studies and reports all show that it supports energy production *inside* of your cells, and is especially important for strong and healthy blood flow which not only helps your heart, but your entire circulatory system.
- In order for CoQ10 to be fully utilized by your body it must be converted into its reduced firm, known as-
- **Ubiquinol:** 95 % of CoQ10 that naturally exists in your body is ubiquinol. Thus, if you take Ubiquinol CoQ10, your body can use it right away. Whereas, if you take ubiquinon CoQ10, your body will need to convert it to ubiquinol before it can use it. There is every possibility that the conversion may not happen effectively.
- For best results for **intra cellular** and **extra cellular** effects, take both.
- As you know Ubiquinol is more absorbable (since the body contains 95% of Ubiquinol) than Ubiquinon. Moreover, ubiquinol and ubiquinone *work well together* - inside AND outside your cells to give you the maximum benefits of CoQ10. Thus, your body needs both forms of CoQ10.
- However, if you can only afford one take Ubiquinol.
- Moreover, with the combined power of ubiquinol and ubiquinone, you'll get amazing results - — so you can keep your heart pumping strong, your blood flowing smooth, and your whole body energized so you feel young and vibrant.
- Remember Coq10 levels declines as you age. While everyone can benefit taking CoQ10 supplements, they are critical specially for people with Cardiovascular conditions and also for those who are taking cholesterol lowering statin drugs which further deplete their CoQ10 levels - otherwise ironically serious heart condition may arise.
- See - *Secretes To Lowering Cholesterol With Nutrition And Natural Supplements, Safely* by Dr. Art T Dash, M.Sc, M>S>, Ph.D., Published by AuthorHouse, 2009.

- Because of your heart's **huge energy requirements,** the need for the potent antioxidant CoQ10 is vital for a healthy heart and cardiovascular system.

Chapter Two

What CoQ10 Deficiency Does To Your Body

Clinical studies have linked significantly decreased levels of CoQ10 to a wide variety of diseases. Because the enzyme CoQ10 is in high concentration in heart muscle cells, deficiency has been linked to cardiovascular diseases, including angina, arrhythmia, heart failure, Problems, such as blood sugar regulation, gum disease, and stomach ulcer have also been linked to CoQ10 deficiency.

Those who are taking cholesterol lowering statins run the risk for COQ10 deficiency, because not only do statins deplete CoQ10 levels, but they also block CoQ10 synthesis in the body. Low CoQ10 levels or deficiency will cause cardiovascular diseases as described above. Furthermore, statin drugs have horrendous side effects such as fatigue, aching joints and muscle cramps, liver and kidney damage, cognitive impairments.

For more information consult my book: *Secretes To Lowering Cholesterol With Nutrition And Natural Supplements, Safely,* by Dr. Art T Dash, M.Sc., M.S., Ph.D. Published By AuthorHouse, 2009.

However. Statin drugs aren't the only culprits,

In fact, there is a long list of pharmaceutical drugs (to name a few, see below) that rob your body of CoQ10. Furthermore, about 50% of American adults take at least one prescription drug daily, it's more imperative than ever to supplement with CoQ10 so you can be sure your body has the necessary levels required for proper cellular energy function and a strong cardiovascular system.

The drugs, Beta Blockers commonly used for the treatment of high blood pressure and arrhythmia, also deplete CoQ10 levels. Some of the psychoactive drugs (e.g., tricyclic antidepressants and phenothiazines) and drugs used to treat arrhythmia, congestive heart failures, and heart attacks also rub the body of CoQ10.

Supplementing CoQ10 will help protect you against the toxicity of these drugs

Chapter Three

Here are some of The Other Uses and Benefits

High Blood Pressure

Numerous clinical studies involving small numbers of people indicate that CoQ10 may reduce blood pressure. But it may take 4 to 12 weeks before you see any effects. In one analysis, researchers reviewed 12 clinical trials which led them to conclude that CoQ10 has the ability to reduce systolic blood pressure by up to 12 mm Hg and diastolic blood pressure by 10 mm Hg without significant side effecys. However, more research involving large number of people is needed. DO NOT self-treat high blood pressure. Discuss with your healthcare provider before you take any steps

High Cholesterol

People with high cholesterol tend to have low levels of CoQ10. Thus, CoQ10 has been suggested as a treatment for high cholesterol, but adequate scientific studies are lacking. However, it may reduce serious side effects from cholesterol lowering statin drugs. These drugs also deplete natural levels of CoQ10 in the body which might cause serious health problems. Thus, supplementing with CoQ10 not only bringing the levels back to normal, but may also help to reduce various side effects associated with stain drug treatment. If you are taking statin drugs, ask your healthcare provider for taking CoQ10 with stains.

For more information consult my book *Secretes To Lowering Cholesterol With Nutrition And Natural Supplements, Safely,* by Dr. Art T Dash, M.Sc., M.S., Ph.D. Published By AuthorHouse, 2009.

Diabetes

Taking CoQ10 may improve heart health and blood sugar problems and help manage high blood pressure in diabetic patients. Preliminary research studies showed that CoQ10 improves blood sugar control. But other studies showed no effect. If you have diabetes consult with your healthcare provider before taking CoQ10.

After Heart Attack

One clinical study reported that people who took daily CoQ10 supplements within 3 days of a heart attack were less likely to have subsequent heart attacks and chest pain. They were also less likely to die of heart disease than those who did not take the supplements. Anyone who has had a heart attack should talk to his/her doctor before taking any herbs or supplements, including CoQ10

Heart Failure

There is a strong link between diminished levels of CoQ10 in patients with heart failure and the severity of reduced pumping function and shortness of breath. A growing body of evidence has emerged showing the benefits of replenishing depleted levels with supplemental CoQ10 in patients with heart failure.

Several clinical studies suggests that CoQ10 supplements help reduce swelling in the legs; reduce fluid in the lungs, making breathing easier; and increase exercise capacity in people with heart failure.

A recently published trial studied of 420 patients with heart failure receiving the best conventional medical therapy: half were randomized to receive CoQ10 and half to placebo. **Over 2 years of follow-up, those taking CoQ10 had 50% fewer "major" heart complications-including 43% fewer deaths.** And this benefit came with no increase in side-effects. In fact, there was a trend toward fewer side-effects in the CoQ10 group than in those taking a placebo!

This finding is corroborated by a recent large review of 13 prior studies that showed an overall benefit in pumping ability of weak heart when treated with CoQ10.

The CoQ10 story is a fascinating one and continues to evolve. If you feel that you might benefit from taking CoQ10, share this information with your health care provider. **Please remember: always consult with your health care provider before changing your prescription medicines in any way or starting a new supplement.**

Heart Surgery

Clinical research study shows that taking CoQ10 prior to heart surgery, including bypass surgery and heart transplantation , can reduce oxidative damage caused by free radicals, strengthen heart function and lower the incidence of irregular heart beat (arrhythmia) during recovery phase. You are advised not to take any supplements before surgery without the approval of your doctor.

Guarding the Brain After Cardiac Arrest

People who survive cardiac arrest often suffer irreversible brain damage as a result of the disruption of oxygen to the brain. European researchers recently investigated whether combining CoQ10 with mild hypothermia—a technique proven to reduce neuronal damage and increase survival—might enhance the effects of that treatment

The patients were then administered either liquid CoQ10 (250 mg followed by 150 mg three times daily for five days) or a placebo through a nasogastric tube. The remarkable findings showed that three-month survival in the CoQ10 group was 68%, compared to only 29% in the placebo group. Coenzyme Q10 thus helped reduce the death rate from cardiac arrest by an astounding 57%. The researchers also found that 36% of patients in the CoQ10 group had a good neurological outcome at three months, versus only 20% in the placebo group.

Helps Slow Neurodegenerative Disease Progression

Several Researchers have conducted preclinical trials examining how oxidative stress and impaired mitochondrial function may contribute to neuronal cell death, a characteristic of Parkinson's, Alzheimer's, and other neurodegenerative diseases. For instance,, a recent article in *Toxicology and Applied Pharmacology Journal* reported on the effects of the herbicide paraquat on neuronal cell death in the laboratory.

The researchers found that this toxic chemical damaged mitochondria and increased free radical production, eventually resulting in neuronal cells death. Pretreatment of the cell cultures with CoQ10, however, inhibited both mitochondrial dysfunction and free radical production. The researchers hypothesized that coenzyme Q10 may prove useful in preventing and treating neurodegenerative conditions related to environmental toxins.

Slows The Progression Of Macular Degeneration

Age related macular degeneration (AMD) is one of the major causes of vision loss in people over 60. With the deterioration of the macula (a tiny cluster of highly specialized cells in the retina) the central vision progressively begins to blur. As the disease worsens, the central vision loss may increase until it becomes impossible to perform daily tasks, such as reading, writing and driving.

Researchers treated the patients with two capsules per day containing 200 mg of acetyl L-carnitine, 780 mg of omega-3 fatty acids, and 20 mg of CoQ10. At the end of 12 month treatment period, they found statistically significant improvements in the treatment group. Only one of the 48 patients in the treatment group showed clinically significant worsening in the vision field.

My recommendation: increase Ubiquinol CoQ10 to100 mg twice daily, and take PQQ 10 mg with CoQ10 only once.

Gum (Periodontal) disease

Gum disease is a common problem that causes swelling, bleeding, pain, and redness of the gums. Clinical studies show that people with gum disease tend to have low levels of CoQ10 in their gums. A few studies with small numbers of people found that CoQ10 supplements led to faster healing and tissue repair, but more research is needed.

LIFE EXTENSION MAGAZINE
CoQ10's "Other" Health Benefits
February 2006
By Sherry Kahn, MPH

Here are some of the other benefits of CoQ10 may

- Improve immune system function in people with HIV or AIDs
- Be effective in the treatment angina, atherosclerosis (hardening of arteries), Arrhythmia, cardiomyopathy, congestive heart failure
- Improve heart muscle cells and repair all our blood vessel walls,
- Be used in the treatment of male fertility, increase sperm motility and sperm counts, other nutrients recommended along with CoQ10 are L-argentine, L-carnitine,
  Vitamins C, E and zinc
- Be used as part of the treatment for Parkinson disease
- **Mitral Valve Prolaps**: this means one of the heart valves is not closing properly as your heart contracts and expands. CoQ10 may alleviate this condition, ideally in combination with magnesium.
  Increase exercise ability in people with angina
- **Muscular Dystrophy**: a group of diseases characterized by progressive muscle weakness.
- CoQ10 improves physical performance and quality of life. Take also L-carnitine
- **Help** prevent migraines

- **Periodontal Disease**: numerous studies have found that CoQ10 can improve the health of Gum. If you have chronic bleeding gum due to gingivitis, you should give CoQ10 a try.
- **But the key to staying young is having MORE mitochondria that are healthy enough to produce energy.**
- **Drug Damage**: several drugs rub the body of CoQ10. For instance, Adriamycin (a chemotherapy drug,) CoQ10 acts as an antioxidant to protect the heart and body from the damaging effects of chemotherapy agents).
- **But when you combine PQQ with CoQ10, amazing things can happen.**

Remember, the more of these **power generators** you have, the more you'll feel like that **energetic 5-year-old** who never seems to run out of steam

Chapter Four

How CoQ10 Helps Fight Cancer

Unlike healthy cells, cancer cells don't die. They are immortal. Cancer cells divide relentlessly forming solid tumors or flooding the blood with abnormal cells. Cancer cells cancer cells keep making copies in an unregulated pace. They can also spread from one part of the body to another in a process known as metastasis. Cancer cells also invade other healthy tissues. Cancer cells hide among the healthy cells by mimicking as healthy cells. As a result, killer cells of the immune system fail to recognize them and destroy them.

Chemotherapy treatment has the same problem. It cannot differentiate cancer cells from healthy cells. Thus, the chemotherapy agents kill cancer cells along with healthy cells. For some reason cancer cells attack and kill mitochondria in heart tissues. Chemotherapy agents produce horrendous side effects causing various chronic health illnesses, including serious heart conditions.

As you have seen from above discussions, CoQ10 energizes mitochondria (power house of cells) in your cells that lead to remarkable effects against common heart ailments and neurological disorders. Lately, scientists have been able to unravel specific mechanism indicating that CoQ10 may play a significant role in fighting certain cancers and improving heart conditions.

Cancer is both the result of and a **leading** cause of free radical damage associated with inflammation. A growing awareness of this significant and intimate link has driven scientists to explore ways of controlling cancer growth by limiting free radical damage.

This line of thinking led us not onl;y to understand how cancer develops, but also of our struggles to limit the horrendous side effects of chemotherapy drugs (anddrialmycin or anthracyclines) on healthy tissues. As it is well known that the antioxidant CoQ10 promotes cardiovascular health and brain health, it is not surprising that the cutting edge medical researchers turned to CoQ10 for possible aid to prevent from the ravages of chemotherapy drugs.

It is even more surprising to note that this versatile nutrient seems to actually increase cancer killing effects of chemotherapy drugs themselves, and also protects the heart from cardiotoxicity. Animal studies showed that CoQ10 could protect against the burst of free radical release resulting from chemotherapy treatment of various cancers.

The researchers focused on CoQ10 and cancer on two vital fronts – CoQ10's ability to increase immune system response and it's ability to reduce the cardiotoxicity caused by a common class of anti-cancer therapeutic agents. They also discovered that cancer patients exhibit low levels of CoQ10.

When CoQ10 was used in combination with chemotherapy drugs, researchers began to observe that CoQ10 was having an independent beneficial impact – it was helping to energize immune system cells that had been suppressed by cancer. It restored their ability to fight back by attacking the cancer cells (it is well known that the immune system is a powerful defense against cancer metastasis.)

Based on this immunostimulatory effect of CoQ10, Danish researchers investigated CoQ10's impacts in combination with other nutrients as an adjunctive therapy for breast cancer. In one research report, the researchers describe three breast cancer patients with metastasized cancer. These women were treated with chemotherapy along with the supplementation of a daily dose of 300 mg of CoQ10. All three women showed tumor regression and decreased incidence of metastasis.

There are other similar studies involving conventional cancer therapy and immunostimulating agents like vitamins C (3000 mg), E (2500 IU) , selenium (387 mcg), beta carotene (25000 IU), omega-3 fatty acids (1.2 grams), of course, CoQ10 (90 mg) and PQQ 10-20 mg, where, at the end of 18 months, patients showed partial remission , none of the patients showed signs of additional metastases, and their quality of life improved. Increasing the dose of CoQ10 to 300 mg, better results were achieved.

The cancer drugs are highly effective; however, they produce serious toxic side effects on heart tissues, possibly leading to cardiomyopathy, and heart failure that are not responsive to conventional pharmacological interventions. In fact, the cancer drug anthracyclines selectively damage mitochondria in heart, but not other organs.

Since CoQ10 supports both heart tissues and mitochondria, researchers conducted human trials to determine if CoQ10 might prevent cardiotoxicity during administration of cancer drug anthracyclines. According to a report in **The Journal of Clinical Oncology**, summarized five reviewed studies in which CoQ10 was given along with anthracyclines

They found that the patients who took CoQ10 showed favorable changes in their heart rhythms suggesting that CoQ10 might have stabilizing effect on the heart. They also note that the supplementation did not interfere with anthracyclines treatment and no adverse effects were reported in any of the trials. Still more rigorous investigations are needed.

Chapter Five

Brain and Heart Need PQQ (pyrroloquinoline quinine)

Supper Star Nutrient PQQ

If you want to stay youthful and have all the benefits and power of youth as long as possible, it is essential to know two very important words: **Telomere and Mitochondria.**

Telomere: Telomeres are the bits of DNA at the ends of each chromosome.

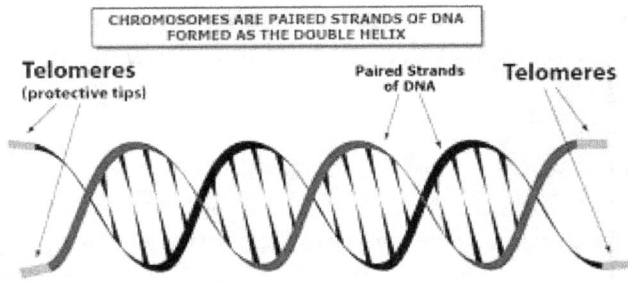

CHROMOSOMES ARE PAIRED STRANDS OF DNA
FORMED AS THE DOUBLE HELIX

Telomeres
(protective tips)

Paired Strands
of DNA

Telomeres

Each time your cells divide, your telomeres shorten. When your telomeres are gone, your cells stop dividing – and die.

Scientists have shown that **by lengthening the telomeres, you should be able to increase your cell's lifespan by enabling them to divide many more times, thereby increasing your life span**

The discussions of telomeres will take us far afield. We will just focus our discussions on mitochondria.

Mitochondria: *The source of life in your body*

MITOCHONDRION

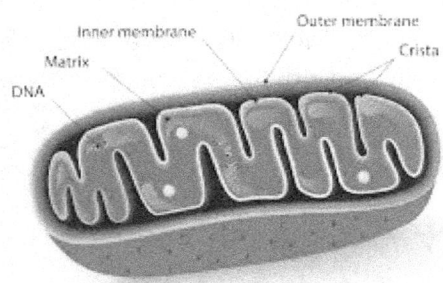

Inner membrane

Outer membrane

Matrix

Crista

DNA

From: 1000x675.redorbit.com

Your mitochondria – tiny power plants that should crackle with energy – combine oxygen, proteins and nutrients, including CoQ10 to make ***adenosine triphosphate*** (ATP).

It has been reported that CoQ10 activates the production of ATP; and CoQ10 resides primarily in inner membranes of the mitochondria. 95 % of all cellular energy production depends on it.

CoQ10 is a nutritional powerhouse for mitochondrial health. Taking CoQ10 supplement helps protect mitochondrial membranes from oxidative damage. This in turn has been helpful for a slew of chronic health disorders and debilitating diseases.

Every second of the day, your mitochondria should pump out this ATP that fuels your cells.

And it should give you the power that fuels your heart, brain and every tissue and cell in your body.

But you need one nutrient to make it all happen... a nutrient your body's running out of... CoQ10. CoQ10 is required for mitochondrial ATP synthesis and functions as an antioxidant in cell membranes.

Cells contain 2 to 2,500 mitochondria depending upon which cells. For instance, each brain cell contains 2000 mitochondria. Thus, without supporting mitochondria your mobility and muscle strength disappear **much faster.**

Mitochondria are the only power plant inside each cell. They are so critical they have their own DNA and that's what connects them to telomeres

Mitochondria have circular chromosomes with a DNA complex that code for 37 genes. This special DNA helps your body generate and manufacture cellular energy.

Like your telomeres this mitochondrial DNA is a marker that indicates how quickly you age

Recently a team of researchers from Johns Hopkins University showed a connection between how much mitochondrial DNA you have in your blood, and how frail and weak you become as you age.

They found that your risk of fraility and muscle weakness go up as the DNA in your mitochondria start to disappear. Furthermore, doctors at John's Hopkins University also found that people with the lowest amount of mitochondrial DNA have a **47 % greater risk of dying from all causes.**

Thus, genes inside your mitochondria are clear indicator of your overall power and strength as you age, and the more you have, the more you feel younger and live longer.

Your cells can have anywhere from 2 to 10,000 mitochondria. Depending on the size of a person, a person may have anywhere from 100 trillion cells in the body. Now you can imagine what an enormous number of mitochondria are in your body.

Unfortunately, mitochondria die off as we get older. That is why the researchers at Johns Hopkins University were able to establish connection between weakness and fraility, and disappearing mitochondria. Thus, you can see why it is so vital to **grow new mitochondria.**

Chapter Six

As Your Mitochondria Disappear, So Does Your Life Force

Mitochondria have their own DNA. That means they can **REPLICATE.** They replicate independently of the cell in which they reside. This means mitochondrial replication is not coupled to cell division. Thus, they INCRESE numbers within a cell, if they have the right nutrient. This nutrient is PQQ, Pyroloquinoline quinine. Researchers proved that PQQ produce **new mitochondria.**

Researchers at the University of California at Davis are pioneers in the study of PQQ. Their work showed a clear connection between PQQ and the growth of new mitochondria

- **PQQ Promotes New Mitochondrial Formation:** recent studies showed the PQQ's unique ability to stimulate the growth of new mitochondria and improve the function of existing mitochondria. This is an important longevity strategy that can help prevent the disease of aging.
- It would be hard to overstate the dramatic impact it has on the entire body, especially the **brain.** PQQ has been shown to protect the brain from neurodegenerative damage, stroke damage, and even the impact of traumatic brain injury. PQQ stimulates the natural production of **nerve**
- **growth factor (NGF)** which triggers the growth of brand new nerve cells and brand new brain cells. New growth factor is required for the development and maintenance of nerve cells, including many of the cells that are vital **for memory, cognition,** and **learning.** NGF is vital in repairing damage caused by stroke.
- **PQQ Protects Brain From Excitotoxicity:** excessive stimulation of brain cells called excitotoxicity is the major factor in the development of long-term neurodegenerative conditions like stroke, and schizophrenia. This overstimulation of brain cells triggers undesired cell death (apoptosis or cell suicide) leading to senility and memory loss as you grow older.
- Fortunately, not only can PQQ help protect against the damaging impacts of excitotoxicity, it can also help prevent from occurring to begin with. PQQ not only generates power plants, but also helps restore younger, faster brain power. All that new energy keeps your heart young too. PQQ's strong antioxidant power helps shield the mitochondria in your heart from the stress of making all that energy.

Chapter Seven

Healthy Brains Need Healthy Mitochondria

Brain is the most energy hungry organ in your body, since your brain cells contain the largest number of mitochondria. More than 2,000 of them in each nerve cell. Thus, healthy brain needs well functioning mitochondria.

In order brain to be healthy, you need well functioning mitochondria. However, as you grow older your mitochondria decay, become weaker and die. As a result, their numbers are reduced. This is a primary cause of aging and also the cause of many neurodegenerative diseases, such as Alzheimer's, Parkinson's and dementia.

Recent clinical studies reveal that your brain is a prime target for mitochondrial decay more than any other organs in your body. This is because of the high-energy demands of your brain cells, and their exposer to large amounts of oxygen makes them vulnerable to damage from free radicals and oxidative stress.

If the damage is too severe, the brain cells trigger the destruction of their own mitochondria. Fewer mitochondria in your brain cells mean you lose your ability to make energy and your mental performance decline.

Ultimately, this causes your brain cells commit "**cell Suicide or apoptosis.**" This loss of cells in your brain tissue affects your **mobility**, your ability to **learn**, and your **memory**, leading **to all kinds of neurological and brain disorders.**

Fortunately we have PQQ to the rescue.

PQQ functions as a neuroprotective agent that can help protect **memory** and **cognition,** and prevents neurodegenerative diseases like Alzheimer's and Parkinson's. PQQ has a restorative and rejuvenating effect on your brain. See the following descriptions.

- Mitochondria have their own supply of DNA. If they are supplied with the super nutrient PQQ.   They start multiplying within each of your cells. It triggers your aging brain cells to grow new   mitochondria, and improves the functions of existing mitochondria.
- PQQ also protects and restores the existing mitochondria in your brain cells by mopping up free   radicals and the oxidative stress damage in brain tissue – these very things that kill mitochondria in the first place
- The cells' microscopic energy factories, the mitochondria manufacture ATP to fuel all life's activities, It is this processes of "mitochondrial biogenesis" that impede and reverses cell death and brain degeneration. PQQ is the only nutrient that can do all this.

Ischemic Stroke:

Ischemic stroke occurs when blood supply to the brain is interrupted or blocked depriving the brain of vital nutrients/oxygen it needs.   This causes **brain cell death.** Strokes can cause paralysis, memory impairments, and even death

PQQ can play a vital role in preventing brain from ravages of strokes. In clinical studies, it was shown that PQQ reduced ischemic stroke damage potentially improving quality of life following a stroke.

Chapter Eight

PQQ Inhibits Malformed Brain Proteins:

One of the major contributing factors in the development of Alzheimer's and Parkinson's diseases is the accumulation of **malformed proteins.** In Alzheimer's, these are collectively referred to as   **beta amyloid.** Beta amyloid proteins cause a great amount of damage and ultimately kill brain cells.

Clinical studies showed that PQQ **reversed** the toxicity of beta amyloid proteins. **Prevented** brain cell death, **reduced** oxidative damage caused by malformed proteins, and revived those cells that had begun to die.

In Parkinson's disease, the abnormal protein deposits in the brain contain tangled fibrils of a protein called **alpha-synuelein** that is toxic to brain tissues. PQQ deters the formation of these cell killing fibrils which helps protect cells from oxidative damage.

Scientists are exceedingly excited about PQQ's ability to inhibit the formation of toxic protein fibrils in both Alzheimer's and Parkinson's diseases.

Chapter Nine

PQQ Prevents Glucose-Induced Brain Damage

Chronic exposure to elevated blood sugar levels may cause serious damage to brain cells. Furthermore, the elevated insulin levels usually associated with diabetes also contribute to the neurological damage.

These facts have convinced many scientists to refer to Alzheimer's disease as Type 3 diabetes.

In clinical studies it has been shown that PQQ can help protect against the damage caused by elevated blood sugar, and elevated insulin levels.

A growing body of evidences suggests that PQQ can help with Alzheimer's disease and Parkinson's disease, as well as increasing memory functions.

- PQQ helps increase sperm motility, improving male fertility

Your mitochondria (your cells energy factories) need CoQ10 to generate ATP energy to keep your heart and brain cells functioning and healthy.
CoQ10 is a critical piece of the puzzle because it acts as the "spark plug" inside your mitochondria. CoQ10 helps each individual mitochondria make energy

Thus, the key to staying young and healthy is having MORE mitochondria that are healthy enough to produce energy.

Remember, the more of these power generators you have, the more you'll feel like that energetic 5-year-old who never seems to run out of steam

Therefore, when you combine PQQ with CoQ10, amazing things can happen.

Chapter Ten

PQQ Induces Cancer Cell Death

In recent study, PQQ has been reported as a most promising cancer fighting agent that might contribute to tumor cell apoptosis and death. PQQ induce tumor cells apoptosis (a cell commit suicide).

Recent studies indicated that PQQ could induce apoptosis in human Promonocytic leukemia U937 and lymphoma EL-4 cells, as well as Jurkat cell programmed death. These findings suggest that PQQ not only regulates redox of the cells, but also poses impacts on cellular signaling pathways [6]

PQQ turns the mitochondria of cancerous cells against themselves by using the microscopic power plant to trigger apoptosis. PQQ also attacks tumors by cutting off or reducing their sources of blood. It also deters the tumors ability to grow new blood vessels.

Moreover, PQQ turns off genes that help promote the spread of cancer and at the same time, it combats cancer causing inflammation.

Researchers at a University of Shanghai, China found that PQQ worked so well at destroying cancer cells with its low toxicity treatment, they recommended its potential use as a wide spread cancer therapy. [5]

PQQ was discovered by a group of Japanese scientists back in 1970. At the time, they did not know the full power and benefits of this nutrient except that it appeared to play some role in ensuring the propagation of our species.

Further research demonstrated the effects of PQQ on the output of energy from mitochondria, the microscopic energy factories inside each of your cells.

Since then further research has indicated several important impacts of PQQ on the body's cellular processes. But the feeling is further research is to be done to unravel its impact on brain, heart, and body.

Study showed that PQQ prevented a number of heart cells self destroying when scientist deprived them of oxygen and glucose. Furthermore, when cells are under stress, PQQ steps up to prevent apoptosis; it sends mitochondria into overdrive to give the cells extra energy so they don't self-destruct under strain.

PQQ plays a vital role in helping the body maintain the delicate balance of cell life and cell death, without it there would be no cell development. If too few cells die, you can develop cancer. If too many cells die, you can suffer a stroke, heart attack, a neurological disease or many other health disorders.

The concept of cell suicide sounds scary, but as you see from above it is absolutely essential to your survival. Your body's cells are dying constantly and are constantly being replaced or replicated. Your very existence depends on this cycle of life, since new cells often undergo slight changes to help them to improve their performance. Cell suicide is programmed into your genes.

Your cells are constantly replicating. Your body today is not the same it was yesterday.

But while PQQ promotes cell life by supercharging your mitochondria, spurring them to duplicate more rapidly, it also uses its cell-suicide function directly against cancer cells. [3,4]

Chapter Eleven

Where is it found the most?

The highest concentrations of PQQ, similar to CoQ10, are **in the power centers of your body,** those which require the most energy, vital organs like the heart, liver, kidneys, spleen, pancreas, there are are also very high concentrations of PQQ in the brain.

Your body does not produce PQQ. You must replenish your body with PQQ from outside sources, that is, taking PQQ supplements. You may also consume foods rich in PQQ, such as

Parsley, green tea, green peppers, papaya, carrot, celery, spinach, Nato, legumes, pava beans, sweet potatoes, apple, kiwi, oranges, peanuts

PQQ has even been discovered in interstellar stardust, which has led some scientists to theorize about its role in the evolution of life on Earth.

The following ways can also improve mitochondria function and enhance energy nd wellness.

PQQ Prevents Bone Loss

As testosterone declines in aging men and decline of estrogen in older women lead to bone loss; and increased risk of fractures in both men and women, respectively. This decline of testosterone in men and deficiency of estrogen in older women may induce osteoporosis in both men and women, respectively.

PQQ is well known for its ability to produce new mitochondria in the heart, brain, other tissues, and cells. You know that mitochondria are tiny power houses in each cell that supply fuel to each cell. Now a clinical study of an animal model (mouse study model) revealed that supplementing with the nutrient PQQ protected bone strength by preventing the decline in bone cell function.

The research showed that PQQ significantly slowed testosterone deficiency related osteoporosis. This means PQQ supplementation may emerge as a **bone restoration** strategy for men. Furthermore, the study demonstrates PQQ's promise to not only protect against bone loss associated with low testosterone, but also to aid in producing healthy **youthful** bones

In the advent of this animal model stuy, it is imperative to anticipate human studies that investigate and confirm these exciting new findings. In the meantime, men and women should consider supplementing (10-20 mg) with PQQ daily along with well-researched bone-forming nutrients, such as calcium, vitamin D3, boron, magnesium, zinc, vitamin K2, and silicon.

The findings from the animal model study provide new indication on strategies to prevent and probably reverse an ailment (osteoporosis) that affects aging men and women.

Reference: Life Extension Magazine, Special Winter Edition, 2017 – 2018.

Eat Less: study shows that caloric restriction extends lifespan. When you cut back on food **fewer demands are made on your mitochondria, and production of damaging free radicals declines**. This not only enhances mitochondrial efficiency, but also turns on SIRT1 genes, which encode proteins that boost cellular function. The result? Better health and a longer life.

Heavy Exercise: tunes up existing mitochondria and activates biochemical pathways that stimulate the production of new ones

resveratrol, which activates SIRT1 genes—the same ones that are turned on by caloric restriction. resveratrol, which activates SIRT1 genes—the same ones that are turned on by caloric restriction. SHRT 1 genes extend life span

Alpha Lipoic acid is also important for promoting mitochondrial biogenesis.

References

1.Xu, F., et al. "Pyrroloquinoline quinone inhibits oxygen-glucose deprivation-induced apoptosis by activating the P13K/AKT pathway in cardiomyocytes." Molecular and Cellular Biochemistry. 2014, January. Volume 386, Issue 1-2, P 107-115..

2. Crow, M.T., et al. "The mitochondrial death pathway and cardiac myocyte apoptosis." Circulation Research. 2004; 95: 957-970. doi: 10.1161/01.RES.0000148632.35500.d9.

3. Stites, T., et al. "Pyrroloquinoline quinone modulates mitochondrial quantity and function in mice." J. Nutr. 2006; 136 (2): 390-6.

4. Zhihui, M., et al. "Pyrroloquinoline quinone induces cancer cell apoptosis via mitochondrial-dependent pathway and down-regulating cellular Bcl-2 protein Expression." Journal of Cancer. 2014; 5(7): 609–624. Published online 2014 Jul 29.doi: 10.7150/jca.9002.

5. Zhihui, M. et al. Ibid.

6. He K, Nukada H, Urakami T, Murphy MP. Antioxidant and pro-oxidant properties of pyrroloquinoline quinone (PQQ): implications for its function in biological systems. Biochemical pharmacology. 2003;65:67–74. [PubMed]

7. Life Extension, April 216

8. Emails From: Drs Al Sears, MD,, Mercola, MD, Julian Whitaker MD, Mark Stengler, America's Naturopath